# Acid Alkaline Diet For Beginners:

## Lose Weight Naturally, Rebalance pH Levels and Improve Health

By

Valerie Alston

# Table of Contents

Introduction .................................................................... 5

Chapter 1. Acidity Level and Health................................ 7

Chapter 2. Effects of Too Much Acid in The Body ............ 11

Chapter 3. Benefits of Properly Alkalized Body ................ 14

Chapter 4. Maintaining pH Balance Through Diet ............. 16

Chapter 5. Alkaline-Promoting Foods ............................... 23

Conclusion ..................................................................... 31

Thank You Page .............................................................. 32

Acid Alkaline Diet For Beginners: Lose Weight Naturally, Rebalance pH Levels and Improve Health

By Valerie Alston

© Copyright 2015 Valerie Alston

Reproduction or translation of any part of this work beyond that permitted by section 107 or 108 of the 1976 United States Copyright Act without permission of the copyright owner is unlawful. Requests for permission or further information should be addressed to the author.

This publication is designed to provide accurate and authoritative information in regard to the subject matter covered. This work is sold with the understanding that the publisher is not engaged in rendering legal, accounting, or other professional services. If legal advice or other expert assistance is required, the services of a competent professional person should be sought.

First Published, 2015

Printed in the United States of America

# Introduction

The mechanisms and operations of the body are guided by a set of homeostatic processes. This state of equilibrium includes a normal balance and blood concentration of various compounds, hormones and enzymes designed to operate optimally at certain blood pH. Although blood and body pH are designed to be slightly alkaline, there are instances when the pH of the blood and of the body are made slightly acidic from various factors such as diet, stress and exposure to pollutants.

This condition cannot be prolonged and must be addressed because if allowed for a long time, it encourages the growth of fungus and various organisms that produce acidic toxins. These toxins can interfere with the normal processes within the body producing more toxins, interfering with body functions, slowing down metabolism and facilitating the growth of cancer cells.

Outlined in this book is the ways in which the pH of the body can be returned to its normal alkaline state. Various foods suggestions as well as alternatives are given in order to produce an alkaline body through diet. There is also suggestion on how to incorporate an alkaline-based diet into one's lifestyle.

This book opens you to a healthy alternative diet and lifestyle, which would help you boost your immune system, lower your chances for some forms of cancer and improve your metabolism.

# Chapter 1. Acidity Level and Health

In order to function properly, the body needs to be in a certain form of chemical balance. This chemical balance results in the blood being slightly basic. In order to function properly such pH level must be maintained. The human body is built with a strong homeostatic mechanism and has great sensitivity to blood pH. Whenever something causes the blood pH to be slightly decreased or increase, the body responds with various processes in order to bring the pH level back to normal.

The body maintains this level of pH because various compounds and enzymes in the body are more stable at this state. Beyond the acceptable pH range, some proteins become denatured or are destroyed and cannot do their functions while some enzymes become deactivated. If this condition is prolonged, death becomes inevitable.

**Weight and acidity**

Studies reveal that weight and the pH level of the blood are connected. In a study conducted investigating the fat and blood acidity connection, it was found out that the body produces fat as a response to an increased acidity in the blood. That means, in order to normalize the acidity within the cells in the body, the body compensates by producing fat cells. Furthermore, based from this, we can deduce that fat cells are actually a response that benefits the body. It could be construed, therefore, that in order to remove fats (and reduce weight), one needs to normalize his acidity level first.

For systems that are incapable of producing fat cells to compensate for the acidity in the blood, the acidity in the blood results to an overall acidic environment in the body particularly in the digestive system. This acidic environment favors the growth of fungi and yeast, which feeds on the food consumed by an individual. A study reveals that this leads to as much as 50% reduction to the nutrients absorbed from food. This has caused people to become thin. With little nutrients absorbed, the body cannot have enough of protein to build and repair cells or assist in the production of various enzymes and hormones, which are used for various functions of the body.

In order for the normal operation of the body to be restored, the pH of the body must be brought into normal range (between 7.38 and 7.42), too.

**Immune System Performance**

When the body is below the comfortable range of pH (when it is slightly acidic), various processes in the body are hampered—including the normal immune response. Furthermore, an acidic environment favors the production of toxins and deprives cells of oxygen. Thus, proteins are poorly digested which causes reactions that lead to allergies.

**Energy level and blood acidity**

One of the most notable manifestations of the acidity of the body is fatigue or lethargy. A slightly acidic body produces numerous toxins, which interfere with the normal mechanism of the absorption of minerals and proteins. Without sufficient supply of these nutrients, the body is unable to reconstruct itself and facilitate cellular division at a rate sufficient to compensate with the demands of an acidic body. This equates to poor energy, low endurance and the inability of the muscles to function well.

**Diabetes and Acidity**

The pancreatic juice released by the pancreas (at 8.8) is one of the most basic compounds synthesized and released within the body. When the body does not have enough calcium ions for it, the body is incapable of producing this juice. When this happens, the body, then, finds it difficult to maintain its usual pH levels resulting in the accumulation of waste products in the insulin receptor sites of each cells. In a normal body, because of the alkaline environment, these waste products are effectively neutralized or are washed off into the bloodstream allowing the sites to be free from insulin response.

## Chapter 2. Effects of Too Much Acid in The Body

The state of having too much acid in the body is called acidosis. Two forms of acidosis occurs in the body: metabolic and respiratory. Metabolic acidosis occurs when there is too much acid or the body produces more acid than usual while respiratory acidosis occurs when the body has less oxygen or has more carbon dioxide in the body. Carbon dioxide is a byproduct of metabolic processes. A body that has problems with the respiratory system cannot get rid of carbon dioxide and take in oxygen. When the body is in acidic state, various illnesses happen in the body:

**Upset Stomach**

One of effects of an acidic body is an upset stomach. People with acidic body feels nauseated and may vomit as a result. Appetite is also decreased and digestion is affected.

**Fatigue and Lethargy**

A healthy body has efficient systems that could produce energy efficiently from the food consumed and from various sources. A body under acidic environment is incapable of generating energy from the foods consumed.

## Respiratory Problems

As one of the consequences of high blood levels of acid, one may feel difficulty in breathing. High levels of carbon dioxide in the blood prompts the body to breath more to eliminate this toxic substance from the body. In severe forms of acidosis, one may sustain health-related problems which could lead to fatal complications.

## Confusion

During acidosis, the body gets insufficient amount of oxygen. Without sufficient amount of oxygen, the neurons cannot function properly. This leads to an unusual feeling of confusion and anxiety. Vertigo caused by acidosis interferes with day-to-day activity and makes it difficult to conduct one's daily task.

## Shock, coma and death

If acidosis persists for a long time, various cells and organs in the body sustain damage, which eventually results to them failing in the end. Acidosis also results to decrease in the blood pressure to a point where the body cannot function normally called a state of shock. This leads to dizziness, profuse sweating, chest pain, restlessness and pale skin. The body who sustains acidosis for a short time can sustain damage long enough that the body can no longer keep up. This eventually leads to coma and death.

# Chapter 3. Benefits of Properly Alkalized Body

The body is naturally designed for peak performance and operation at certain levels of pH. When this pH is altered to something less than that of the ideal range, the body begins to fall into disarray. Consequently, when this normal pH range is restored, they body begins to enter a reparative state were the body is restored to its normal functions from the cellular level.

The following are some of the benefits of a properly alkalized body:

**a) Greater resistance against common cold.** An acidic environment promotes the growth of yeast, fungi and bad bacteria. Furthermore, the immune function is weakened or diminished during this state. Thus, the body is unable to fight infections even the minor ones. The body, on the other hand, when in alkalized state promotes the growth of good bacteria thus limiting or keeping the population of bad bacteria in check. The performance of the immune system is also bolstered thereby enabling the body to resist infection more.

**b) Helps prevent cancer.** If the body is acidic, oxygen absorption and utilization drops thereby slowing down or stopping metabolic processes. This condition leads to the growth of cancer cells. An alkalized body, however, facilitates healthy cell turnover, which is the key to cancer prevention.

**c) Healthy weight.** As demonstrated previously, the acidity of the body greatly influences fat storage and weight management. Fruits and vegetables are among the foods that are capable of restoring the normal slightly-basic state of the body. Processed foods, however, containing refined carbohydrates, simple sugar and alcohol tend to nudge the body into a harmful acidic state. It is a established fact that even without the application of the principles of acidity and alkalinity, fruits and vegetables, which are sources of fiber, nutrients and complex carbohydrates are instrumental in maintaining a healthy weight. Foods that are high in calories from carbohydrates, on the other hand, tend to slow down the metabolism, causes hunger and craving and results to obesity in the end.

# Chapter 4. Maintaining pH Balance Through Diet

Although there are, many factors that could affect the acidity of the blood, the food and fluids that we consume (being included in those factors) are among those which we could control. To ensure a proper pH balance, one should do the following:

**Divert from the Usual Breakfast**

Breakfast is the most important meal of the day because it is the meal after eight hours of fasting. That does not mean, however, that your first meal of the day should be filled with sugary foods, however. Examples of the usual foods eaten during breakfast that could increase the acidity of the blood are carbohydrate foods such as breakfast cereals, toast, pancakes muffins, waffles, sweet rolls, honey, orange juice, coffee and muffins.

**Load up on Yellow and Dark Green Vegetables**

Not only are these vegetables rich in dietary fiber which helps flush out toxins from the intestines and help slow down the absorption of carbohydrates, they are also rich in antioxidants, vitamins and minerals which causes the body to achieve a slightly alkaline state—its normal state. Furthermore, they are good sources of alkaline salts that has antifungal, antibacterial and antimycotoxic properties. In addition, chlorophyll, which is considered to be plant's blood are abundant in leafy vegetables which cleanses the body of toxins and impurities. Lastly, green foods (e.g. barley grass and wheat grass) are among the foods with high nutrient value yet with the lowest caloric and sugar content. You can include them in salads or, for convenience and for easy consumption, in the form of juice.

**Prefer low carb vegetables, grains and legumes**

Although they are complex because the carbohydrates are mixed in with other nutrients making every gram of food valuable than refined versions, still, complex carbohydrates are extremely acidifying. Experts agree that foods should contain only as much as 20% of complex carbohydrates and that they should be eaten in moderation. To keep the percentage of carbohydrates at these safe levels, consider low carbohydrate vegetables such as celery, cucumber, eggplant, cabbage, Brussel sprouts, spinach, kale lettuce, onions, okra, green peppers, squash, garlic, parsley and radish. To gauge the quality of a complex carbohydrate, use its color as a reference. The brighter the color is, the more nutrient a carbohydrate vegetable contains. As for legumes, ensure that you consume only fresh legumes as much as possible since stored ones can contain mycotoxins and breeds fungi. Even stored grains should be avoided as molds and fungi which produce mycotoxins tend to grow on them over time. The ideal storage conditions for this are dry and cold temperature with air as dry as possible to discourage the growth of molds. If these conditions are not met, then do not consider eating stored grains if there are still alternatives.

**Feast of sprouts**

The more mature a sprout is the greater are their alkaline properties. Make it a habit to grow and include sprouts in your daily diet. Not only are they easy to grow (they can be easily grown in the kitchen at any season); they are also biogenic foods which means that they tend to transfer their life energy to us.

**Increase the consumption of alkali-forming foods and reduce the consumption of acid-forming foods**

Alkali-forming foods can be as tasty and delectable as the (junk) acid-forming foods when prepared correctly. Since they are fast and easy sources of energy, our body tend to have a taste for them. Gradually, however, as you move your system towards a more alkali-based one, you will develop a taste for alkali-forming foods. One of the best way to take advantage of the substances and nutrients in the vegetables that could encourage alkaline state is to resort to juicing. Juicing breaks down every cell of the plant material into its simplest component that are easily absorbed and used by body. Juicing affords you the benefit you can get from plants minus the taste you are not used to yet. Overtime, as you develop a taste for it, you can combine eating vegetables with juicing. On the other hand, you should avoid foods that form acid in the body such as those derived from animals, dairy products, refined starch and grains and most fruits, which have high concentrations of sugar.

**Be wary with your sources of protein**

Protein is vital in daily operations of the body in its reparative and restorative operations. However, proteins derived from animals are mostly acid forming. The protein that our body requires for optimum performance can be met by vegetables since the protein from animal sources is usually more than our needs. Although it is not advisable that we eradicate animal foods totally from our diet, it should be wiser to minimize them, however.

**Replace water with Alkaline water**

Water is the nutrient humans need constantly. It is said that humans can go on for days without food but is incapable of survival without water for 3 days (at most). Purified water is completely neutral at a pH of 7. Some forms of water are made acidic by some dissolved minerals. Neutral water, however, can be made alkaline by dissolving various form of concentrated solutions or salts available in the market today. If you are serious with consuming Alkaline water, you can invest on home machines which converts normal water into its Alkaline form.

**Eliminate Yeast Containing Foods**

This may not sound altogether appealing to you since most delicious foods are made with yeast such as muffins, pies, cakes, pastries and bread. Studies of countries, which load up on yeast-containing foods, have had high correlations with the prevalence of breast cancer. In comparison, countries which does not have a high consumption of yeast-containing foods such as Japan has lower incidence of the disease. Although the results are still inconclusive, still the correlations suggested by the study are alarming. Furthermore, the correlations

**Eliminate Dairy Products**

Milk has hidden sugars in the form of lactose and contains yeast, fungus, molds and mycotoxins, which can compromise one's health. Lactose is one of the substances that can feed the fungus in the body. Loading up with dairy products and lactose-containing foods is unwise as it can encourage the growth of these toxin producing organisms that can further put the body into acidic state and meddle with the bodies various homeostatic processes.

## Eliminate or limit Fungus foods

They contain mycotoxins which are detrimental to health. There is no such thing as a good mushroom only those with little amounts of toxins that has no observable and immediate effects on the body. The truth, however, is that on molecular levels, the body gradually sustains damage from its ingestion which can be manifested later through diseases after the body has sustained a considerable amounts of damage already.

## Refrain from Alcoholic Beverages

Wines and alcoholic beverages such as beers, whiskey rum, vodka, gin and brandy are produced with the interaction of anaerobic microorganisms that produce mycotoxins as metabolites. They must be avoided at all cost because they do not only add burden to each cells and organs such as the brain, lungs, kidneys and liver but they also cause the system to be acidic which favor the growth of fungi and organisms that produce more mycotoxins.

# Chapter 5. Alkaline-Promoting Foods

A body which is acidic can be prone to various diseases especially if left untreated for a long time. The body can be returned to normal, state, however, with simple tweaks. Here are a list of foods that can be consumed to restore the body to the normal pH:

**Almonds and its milk**

Instead of dairy products, you can opt for more healthy almonds milk as a substitute. Almonds milk are not only better alternatives but brings with them a roster of good effects, too. Because of its high protein content, the food is associated with increased muscle mass, lower cholesterol levels and fat loss. Almonds need not be consumed in large quantities in order for you to benefit from it. You only need to include it in your diet. Additionally, each 100-gram serving contains 27% Calcium, 25% iron and 44% protein.

**Amaranth**

This unfamiliar grain is filled with alkaline forming compounds as well as high quality protein. There are plenty of recipes available online to help you prepare for delicious meal with this alkaline-forming grain.

## Artichokes

Not only are artichokes perfect for salads and as an ingredient in dip, they are also best included in diets and dishes. Artichokes increase the body's pH levels, neutralize, and remove acidic toxins. Artichokes are rich in antioxidants, which are used to clean the liver and aids in digestion. They are best included in salads with green leafy vegetables.

## Arugula

Because of this vegetable's ability to neutralize toxins and acidic compounds, it is usually included in a detox program and diet. This food is filled with alkaline-producing beta-carotene, which has antioxidant properties, too. This product is rich in calcium which makes it an ideal calcium-rich substitute to dairy products.

## Asparagus

When it comes to food that can neutralize body's acidity, nothing beats asparagus. In addition, it has strong antioxidant properties, rich in nutrients and is an excellent detoxifier. Some even notes the anti-ageing properties of this vegetables, which makes this vegetables a nice addition to the menu.

**Avocado & avocado oil**

Avocadoes are considered superfoods because of their high potassium content and healthy fat. This food can make the body alkaline in addition to its cholesterol-lowering effect.

**Basil**

Even spices can have a great effect on the ability of the food to acidify or alkalize the body. Basil is one of the alkaline-producing spices which contain flavonoids which assist the body's natural healing process.

**Beetroot**

Beetroots are good sources of phytonutrient betalain, which has anti-cancer effects. This is one of the foods that can effectively raise the blood's pH restoring its natural alkaline properties. You can include this into your foods as side dish or you can steam it.

**Broccolli**

Brocolli is a rich source of the alkaline form of Vitamin C as well as calcium (highly alkalizing) and vitamin A. Broccolli is an essential addition to a diet if you want to maintain an alkaline body.

**Brussels Sprout**

Brussel sprouts are one of the healthiest of the vegetables. They have been observed to neutralize pH levels of the body and the neutralize various toxic compounds in the body. They contain a variety of nutrients with particularly high percentage of vitamin C.

**Buckwheat**

This food can be used as a gluten-free substitute for most foods that are usually prepared with wheat. Alkalizing versions of buckwheat noodles can be an alternative to the usual acidifying and high-carbohydrate ones. Furthermore, buckwheat has high fiber, iron, calcium and protein contents making this an ideal low-calorie, gluten-free and alkalizing alternative.

**Cabbage**

There are a number of delicious recipes that would enable you to benefit from the alkalizing effect of this vegetable. Because of its alkaline properties, cabbage has been shown to have anti-cancer effects in addition to its high fiber content and low caloric load.

**Carrots**

Carrots are not only good for the eyes and skin because of its high beta carotene contents. They can be consumed raw or added to various food preparations. They are particularly high in Vitamin A, fiber, potassium and other compounds that can neutralize body's acidity.

**Cauliflower**

This vegetable is a source of alkaline version of vitamin C which is more bioavailable than the acidic form. It is easy to prepare an can neutralize various acidic compounds and toxins in the body which makes this a good addition to salads.

### Celery

Celery may not taste good but it is the most alkaline of the vegetables and has low calories. There are many preparations that could render the taste of this food bearable. You can pulverize it, make it into a smoothie or add it to some foods and salads.

### Chia

These seeds have a lot of benefits. They have particularly high pH and can normalize the body's pH in no time. This can be added in soups or added to smoothie.

### Chives.

It is high time that you add chives to your food because they are among the many vegetables that has healing properties and could normalize ones pH. You can be added to various dishes and are good at flavoring up various meal.

### Cilantro

This small leaves can normalize the body's pH in no time. Not only can these leaves normalize the pH, they can also lower the cholesterol and can aid to digestion.

**Coconut**

Fresh coconuts are good sources of healthy fatty acids and are surprisingly highly alkaline. Coconut itself can be eaten raw because they are tasty. They can also be added to foods and can add flavor to most foods.

**Collard Green**

The secret to pH normalizing food is the color. The greener the food is, the more is its ability to neutralize acidity. This vegetable is high in Vitamin A, can neutralize acidity and can help stave off cancer.

**Cucumber**

This is the usual part of salads and can be made into delicious pickled cucumber. This has high alkalizing properties and are best included in various dishes and recipes.

**Cumin**

There are only small list of spices in the world that are capable of keeping the body in alkaline state. Most spices are acidic and can cause the body to assume an acidic state. Cumin is one of those that you could use to flavor your food without the acidic effects. Next time you go for shopping, try to add this to your card and use it to your food. This can neutralize not only the acidity in your body but some of the acidic ingredients in foods, as well.

**Eggplant**

Eggplant is one of the most versatile vegetables in the market. Not only is it good in various dishes but has excellent alkalizing effects as well.

## Conclusion

You just finished reading about the ways on how to tweak your diet in order to achieve an alkaline state or body. The hosts of health benefits are upon you now. Gone were the days for poor food choices and acidic body.

The next step is to incorporate what you learned from this into your lifestyle and allow the information you gained to guide you in choosing healthy food alternatives. If you lead an alkaline based lifestyle, you will gradually notice the changes and the benefits as you will gain more energy and more resistance towards stress. Your immune system will be boosted, too, which will give you the ability to resist certain forms of diseases and to recover from them easily.

Thank You Page

I want to personally thank you for reading my book. I hope you found information in this book useful and I would be very grateful if you could leave your honest review about this book. I certainly want to thank you in advance for doing this.

If you have the time, you can check my other books too.

www.ingramcontent.com/pod-product-compliance
Lightning Source LLC
LaVergne TN
LVHW021745060526
838200LV00052B/3478